Shattered Bonds: The Lingering Shadows of Divorce

Book Introduction:

Shattered Bonds: The Lingering Shadows of Divorce is a comprehensive guide that delves into the complex emotions experienced during the process of divorce. Divorce is an incredibly challenging time, filled with heartache, uncertainty, and upheaval. This book aims to shed light on the tumultuous journey, offering insights, guidance, and support to those who find themselves in the midst of this difficult transition.

In Shattered Bonds, we explore the emotional roller coaster that accompanies divorce. From the initial decision to separate to the aftermath of rebuilding lives, every step of the way presents unique challenges. Divorce not only affects the couple directly involved but also leaves an indelible impact on their children.

Throughout these pages, we emphasize the importance of putting aside personal emotions and focusing on co-parenting for the sake of the children. It is crucial to create an environment where children feel loved, supported, and shielded from the negative consequences of a broken marriage.

This book combines practical advice, psychological insights, and real-life stories to provide a comprehensive resource for navigating the complex landscape of divorce. We address key issues such as legal proceedings, co-parenting challenges, financial considerations, and the long-term effects on emotional well-being. By understanding and acknowledging the lingering shadows of divorce, we can begin the healing process and build a brighter future for ourselves and our children.

Chapter 1: The Decision to Separate

Divorce is not a decision taken lightly. It is often the culmination of months or even years of inner turmoil, unhappiness, and failed attempts at reconciliation. Chapter 1 of Shattered Bonds explores the process of making the decision to separate.

Within these pages, we delve into the emotional struggles faced by individuals who contemplate divorce. We examine the signs of an irreparable relationship, the impact of constant conflict on mental health, and the importance of self-reflection.

Furthermore, we provide guidance on seeking professional help, such as couples' therapy or marriage counseling, as a means to explore all avenues before finalizing the decision to separate. We discuss the significance of clear communication, expressing needs and concerns, and the exploration of alternative solutions.

This chapter aims to offer support and guidance to those who are grappling with the overwhelming choice of ending a marriage. By providing a compassionate and understanding perspective, we strive to empower individuals to make informed decisions and pave the way for a healthier, happier future.

Chapter 2: Navigating the Legal Process

Once the decision to separate has been made, the journey through the legal process begins. Chapter 2 of Shattered Bonds focuses on providing guidance and information on navigating the complex legal aspects of divorce.

Within these pages, we explore the different types of divorce proceedings, including contested and uncontested divorces, and the implications of each. We delve into the role of attorneys and how to find the right legal representation that aligns with your needs and goals.

This chapter also sheds light on important legal considerations such as property division, alimony, child custody, and child support. We discuss the factors that influence these decisions, the legal requirements involved, and strategies for negotiating fair settlements.

Understanding the legal process is crucial for minimizing stress and uncertainty during divorce. We provide a step-by-step breakdown of the legal proceedings, from filing the initial paperwork to attending court hearings. By equipping readers with knowledge about their rights and responsibilities, we aim to empower them to make informed decisions throughout the process.

Additionally, we address the emotional impact that the legal process can have on individuals going through a divorce. From courtroom etiquette to managing emotions during negotiations, we provide practical advice on maintaining composure and advocating for one's best interests.

Navigating the legal process can be overwhelming, but with the guidance and information provided in this chapter, readers will gain the tools they need to approach their divorce proceedings with confidence and clarity.

Chapter 3: Emotional Turmoil: Dealing with Grief and Loss

Divorce is often accompanied by a profound sense of grief and loss. In Chapter 3 of Shattered Bonds, we delve into the emotional turmoil that arises during the process of divorce and offer strategies for coping with these intense feelings.

Within these pages, we acknowledge the range of emotions experienced during divorce, including sadness, anger, fear, and confusion. We emphasize the importance of allowing oneself to grieve the loss of the relationship and the future that was once envisioned.

This chapter explores various coping mechanisms and self-care practices that can aid in navigating the emotional roller coaster of divorce. We delve into the power of self-reflection, mindfulness, and seeking support from friends, family, or professional counselors. We also discuss the potential benefits of joining support groups or engaging in therapeutic activities such as journaling or art therapy.

Furthermore, we address the significance of setting boundaries and establishing a support network to lean on during this challenging time. Learning to prioritize self-care and engage in activities that bring joy and healing can contribute to the process of emotional recovery.

In addition, we provide guidance on effective communication and conflict resolution, particularly when co-parenting is involved. By learning healthy ways to express emotions and engage in constructive dialogue, individuals can foster an environment that is conducive to the well-being of both themselves and their children.

By understanding and addressing the emotional turmoil that accompanies divorce, readers will gain valuable insights and practical tools to navigate their own journey of healing and transformation.

One of the most significant aspects of divorce is the impact it has on children. In Chapter 4 of Shattered Bonds, we explore the challenges and importance of prioritizing the well-being of children throughout the process of co-parenting.

Within these pages, we emphasize the significance of maintaining open lines of communication with your ex-spouse for the sake of the children. We discuss the benefits of establishing a co-parenting plan that outlines responsibilities, visitation schedules, and guidelines for decision-making regarding the children's upbringing.

This chapter delves into the emotional and psychological effects of divorce on children, including feelings of confusion, guilt, and divided loyalty. We provide guidance on fostering a supportive and nurturing environment that allows children to express their emotions and navigate the changes in their lives.

Additionally, we address common co-parenting challenges such as differences in parenting styles, disagreements on major decisions, and conflicts that may arise between parents. We offer practical strategies for effective co-parenting, including active listening, compromise, and finding common ground for the well-being of the children.

Moreover, we explore the importance of maintaining consistency and stability in the children's lives, especially during transitions between households. We discuss strategies for successful co-parenting communication, including the use of technology, shared calendars, and respectful exchanges.

By putting children first and focusing on their needs and best interests, parents can minimize the negative impact of divorce and create a healthy co-parenting dynamic that supports the children's well-being and emotional development.

Chapter 5: Rebuilding Trust and Communication

Divorce can shatter trust and communication between former partners, making it difficult to navigate the post-divorce landscape. In Chapter 5 of Shattered Bonds, we explore the essential process of rebuilding trust and fostering effective communication.

Within these pages, we acknowledge the pain and hurt that may have accumulated during the divorce process. We provide insights into the importance of acknowledging these emotions and working towards forgiveness, both for oneself and one's ex-partner.

This chapter delves into the concept of effective communication as a foundation for successful co-parenting and post-divorce interactions. We discuss strategies for active listening, assertive expression of needs and boundaries, and conflict resolution techniques that can help facilitate healthier conversations.

Rebuilding trust after a divorce can be challenging, but we offer practical steps to establish trust in co-parenting relationships and other areas of life. We emphasize the significance of consistency, honesty, and follow-through in rebuilding trust over time.

Furthermore, we explore the potential for personal growth and self-discovery during the process of rebuilding trust. By focusing on self-improvement and self-compassion, individuals can cultivate healthier relationships with others, including their co-parent.

In this chapter, we also address the importance of setting realistic expectations and boundaries in post-divorce relationships. We provide insights into recognizing and managing potential triggers that may hinder progress in rebuilding trust and communication.

By committing to the journey of rebuilding trust and communication, individuals can lay the groundwork for healthier relationships and a more positive co-parenting experience for the well-being of themselves and their children.

Chapter 6: The Impact of Divorce on Children

Divorce has a profound impact on children, and in Chapter 6 of Shattered Bonds, we delve into the effects divorce can have on children's emotional well-being, development, and overall adjustment.

Within these pages, we explore the range of emotions that children may experience during and after a divorce, including sadness, anger, confusion, and anxiety. We discuss the importance of creating a safe and supportive environment where children feel heard, validated, and reassured.

This chapter addresses the different developmental stages and age groups, highlighting how divorce can affect children at various points in their lives. We provide insights into understanding and responding to children's reactions and behaviors based on their developmental needs.

Additionally, we discuss strategies for open and honest communication with children about divorce, taking into account their level of understanding and providing age-appropriate explanations. We emphasize the importance of maintaining consistent routines, stability, and a sense of belonging for children amidst the changes brought about by divorce.

Furthermore, we explore the potential long-term effects of divorce on children's academic performance, social relationships, and self-esteem. We offer guidance on supporting children through these challenges and fostering resilience in the face of adversity.

In this chapter, we also address the significance of co-parenting cooperation and minimizing conflict in front of children. By providing a united front and demonstrating respect and collaboration, parents can create a more stable and nurturing environment for their children to thrive in.

By understanding the impact of divorce on children and implementing strategies to support their emotional well-being, parents can mitigate the negative effects and help their children navigate the challenges of divorce with resilience and strength.

Chapter 7: Managing Stress and Self-Care

Divorce is an inherently stressful and challenging experience, and in Chapter 7 of Shattered Bonds, we explore the importance of managing stress and prioritizing self-care during this tumultuous time.

Within these pages, we delve into the various sources of stress that can arise during divorce, including legal proceedings, financial concerns, co-parenting challenges, and emotional turmoil. We provide insights into the physical and mental health implications of chronic stress and offer strategies for effectively managing and reducing stress levels.

This chapter emphasizes the significance of self-care as a means of nurturing one's well-being amidst the difficulties of divorce. We discuss the importance of self-compassion, setting boundaries, and engaging in activities that promote relaxation and rejuvenation.

We explore different self-care practices such as exercise, mindfulness, meditation, journaling, and seeking support from friends and family. By taking time for self-reflection and self-care, individuals can replenish their emotional reserves and better cope with the demands of divorce.

Furthermore, we address the importance of seeking professional help, such as therapy or counseling, as a valuable resource for managing stress and emotional well-being. We discuss the potential benefits of professional guidance in navigating the challenges of divorce and healing from its emotional impact.

In this chapter, we also explore the significance of social support and building a network of understanding and empathetic individuals who can provide emotional support during this difficult time. We emphasize the importance of reaching out for help when needed and not carrying the burden alone.

By prioritizing stress management and self-care, individuals can cultivate resilience, reduce the negative impact of divorce-related stress, and promote their overall well-being as they navigate through the complexities of divorce.

Chapter 8: Financial Considerations and Division of Assets

Divorce brings about significant financial considerations, and in Chapter 8 of Shattered Bonds, we explore the importance of understanding and navigating the financial aspects of divorce, including the division of assets and financial planning for the future.

Within these pages, we delve into the various financial considerations that arise during divorce, including property division, spousal support, child support, and financial obligations. We discuss the importance of gathering and organizing financial information, including assets, debts, income, and expenses, to ensure a fair and equitable division.

This chapter provides insights into the different methods of property division, such as equitable distribution or community property, depending on the jurisdiction. We explore strategies for negotiation and settlement to achieve a mutually acceptable resolution.

Additionally, we discuss the significance of financial planning for the post-divorce future. We address topics such as budgeting, managing debts, establishing credit, and securing financial stability. We provide guidance on seeking professional advice, such as consulting with a financial planner or accountant, to make informed decisions about financial matters.

Furthermore, we explore the potential tax implications of divorce and the importance of understanding how divorce may impact income tax filings, exemptions, and deductions. We provide an overview of tax considerations to help individuals navigate this aspect of their financial landscape.

In this chapter, we emphasize the importance of maintaining financial independence and ensuring one's financial security in the aftermath of divorce. We discuss strategies for rebuilding credit, pursuing educational or career opportunities, and establishing financial goals for the future.

By understanding the financial considerations and planning for the future, individuals can navigate the division of assets and financial aspects of divorce with confidence and lay the groundwork for a stable financial future.

Chapter 9: Embracing Change and Rediscovering Identity

Divorce marks a significant turning point in one's life, and in Chapter 9 of Shattered Bonds, we explore the transformative power of embracing change and rediscovering one's identity after divorce.

Within these pages, we delve into the concept of personal growth and self-discovery that can arise from the challenges of divorce. We encourage individuals to view divorce as an opportunity for reinvention and to embrace the changes that come with it.

This chapter addresses the importance of self-reflection and introspection as a means of rediscovering one's values, passions, and aspirations. We provide insights into exploring new hobbies, interests, or career paths that may have been put on hold during the marriage.

Additionally, we discuss the significance of self-empowerment and cultivating a positive mindset during this transitional period. We offer strategies for building self-esteem, practicing self-care, and fostering a sense of purpose and fulfillment.

Furthermore, we explore the potential for personal and interpersonal growth through self-improvement and self-compassion. We discuss the importance of setting boundaries, nurturing healthy relationships, and engaging in personal development activities that foster growth and resilience.

In this chapter, we also address the potential challenges of co-parenting and navigating post-divorce relationships. We offer insights into maintaining healthy boundaries, effective communication, and fostering a positive co-parenting dynamic for the well-being of both parents and children.

By embracing change and rediscovering one's identity, individuals can find strength, purpose, and new possibilities in the aftermath of divorce. This chapter serves as a guide to inspire and support individuals on their journey of self-discovery and personal transformation.

Chapter 10: Creating a New Vision for the Future

Divorce signifies the end of one chapter and the beginning of another. In Chapter 10 of Shattered Bonds, we explore the process of creating a new vision for the future and embracing the opportunities that lie ahead.

Within these pages, we delve into the importance of setting goals and envisioning a fulfilling and purposeful future. We encourage individuals to reflect on their values, aspirations, and dreams, and to use this newfound freedom to chart a path that aligns with their authentic selves.

This chapter addresses the significance of goal setting and creating a roadmap for personal and professional success. We provide insights into establishing short-term and long-term goals, breaking them down into actionable steps, and celebrating milestones along the way.

Additionally, we discuss the importance of self-belief and resilience in pursuing new endeavors. We offer strategies for overcoming self-doubt and fear of the unknown, emphasizing the transformative power of embracing change and taking calculated risks.

Furthermore, we explore the potential for personal and spiritual growth during this transitional period. We discuss the importance of self-reflection, self-acceptance, and cultivating a sense of gratitude and mindfulness as individuals embark on their new journey.

In this chapter, we also address the significance of building a supportive network of friends, family, and mentors who can provide encouragement and guidance during this transformative time. We explore the potential for new and meaningful connections that can enhance the quality of one's life post-divorce.

By creating a new vision for the future, individuals can reclaim their sense of purpose, find joy and fulfillment, and build a life that reflects their truest selves. This chapter serves as a guide to inspire and empower individuals as they embark on this exciting new chapter of their lives.

Chapter 11: Nurturing Healthy Relationships

After divorce, nurturing healthy relationships becomes essential for personal well-being and growth. In Chapter 11 of Shattered Bonds, we explore the importance of fostering positive connections with family, friends, and potential romantic partners.

Within these pages, we delve into the significance of maintaining strong bonds with family members, especially when children are involved. We provide insights into effective co-parenting relationships, building trust, and promoting open communication for the well-being of everyone involved.

This chapter addresses the importance of friendship and building a supportive network of friends who understand and empathize with the challenges of divorce. We discuss strategies for cultivating new friendships, nurturing existing ones, and seeking support during difficult times.

Additionally, we explore the potential for new romantic relationships after divorce. We provide guidance on navigating the dating scene, setting healthy boundaries, and ensuring emotional readiness before entering a new relationship.

Furthermore, we discuss the importance of self-love and self-care as the foundation for nurturing healthy relationships. We emphasize the significance of cultivating a positive self-image, practicing self-compassion, and engaging in activities that promote personal growth and well-being.

In this chapter, we also address the potential challenges that may arise in forming new relationships, such as trust issues, fear of vulnerability, and managing expectations. We offer insights into effective communication, conflict resolution, and maintaining healthy boundaries in both platonic and romantic relationships.

By nurturing healthy relationships, individuals can create a supportive and fulfilling social network that enhances their overall well-being. This chapter serves as a guide to inspire individuals to prioritize connection, foster meaningful relationships, and create a strong support system as they move forward in their post-divorce journey.

Chapter 12: Healing Emotional Wounds

Divorce can leave deep emotional wounds that require healing and growth. In Chapter 12 of Shattered Bonds, we explore the process of healing emotional wounds and finding inner peace after the turmoil of divorce.

Within these pages, we delve into the importance of acknowledging and processing the emotions that arise from divorce, such as grief, anger, sadness, and resentment. We offer insights into healthy coping mechanisms, such as therapy, support groups, and self-reflection, to facilitate emotional healing.

This chapter addresses the significance of self-compassion and self-forgiveness as crucial steps in the healing process. We discuss the power of letting go of blame and embracing forgiveness, both for oneself and one's ex-partner, as a means of releasing emotional burdens and finding inner peace.

Additionally, we explore the potential for growth and personal transformation through self-discovery and self-care. We discuss strategies for nurturing emotional well-being, such as practicing mindfulness, engaging in creative outlets, and exploring new passions or hobbies.

Furthermore, we address the importance of setting boundaries and protecting emotional well-being during the post-divorce journey. We provide insights into recognizing toxic relationships or situations and establishing healthy boundaries to prevent further emotional harm.

In this chapter, we also discuss the potential impact of divorce on self-esteem and self-worth. We offer guidance on rebuilding a positive self-image, fostering self-acceptance, and cultivating a sense of worthiness independent of past relationship experiences.

By embarking on the journey of healing emotional wounds, individuals can find closure, reclaim their emotional well-being, and create a foundation for a brighter and more fulfilling future. This chapter serves as a guide to inspire and support individuals as they navigate the path of emotional healing and growth after divorce.

Chapter 13: Embracing Single Parenthood

In Chapter 13 of Shattered Bonds, we explore the unique journey of embracing single parenthood and navigating the challenges and joys that come with raising children on one's own.

Within these pages, we delve into the importance of embracing the role of a single parent with resilience and determination. We provide insights into the adjustments that need to be made, both practically and emotionally, to provide a stable and loving environment for children.

This chapter addresses the significance of establishing routines, setting boundaries, and maintaining open lines of communication with children. We offer strategies for managing the responsibilities of parenting single-handedly while still finding time for self-care and personal growth.

Additionally, we discuss the importance of seeking support from friends, family, and support groups specifically designed for single parents. We explore the potential for building a strong network of support, sharing experiences, and accessing resources that can alleviate some of the challenges of single parenthood.

Furthermore, we address the potential emotional impact on children growing up in a single-parent household. We provide guidance on fostering a positive and nurturing environment, addressing children's feelings and concerns, and promoting their overall well-being.

In this chapter, we also discuss the importance of self-compassion and self-care for single parents. We emphasize the significance of taking time for oneself, seeking help when needed, and recognizing that it is okay to prioritize personal well-being alongside parenting responsibilities.

By embracing single parenthood with love, patience, and resilience, individuals can provide a nurturing and supportive environment for their children. This chapter serves as a guide to inspire and empower single parents as they navigate the joys and challenges of raising children on their own.

Chapter 14: Moving Forward with Confidence

In Chapter 14 of Shattered Bonds, we explore the transformative power of moving forward with confidence and embracing a future filled with possibilities and personal growth.

Within these pages, we delve into the importance of letting go of the past and embracing the present moment. We provide insights into the power of reframing one's perspective, focusing on gratitude, and finding silver linings in life's challenges.

This chapter addresses the significance of self-belief and self-empowerment as individuals embark on their post-divorce journey. We discuss strategies for building self-confidence, setting achievable goals, and celebrating personal achievements along the way.

Additionally, we explore the potential for personal and professional growth through career advancement, educational opportunities, and pursuing passions that may have been put on hold during the marriage. We discuss the importance of taking calculated risks and stepping outside of one's comfort zone to unlock new opportunities.

Furthermore, we address the potential for new beginnings in various aspects of life, including romantic relationships, hobbies, and personal aspirations. We provide guidance on embracing change, remaining open to new experiences, and finding joy in the pursuit of one's dreams.

In this chapter, we also discuss the importance of practicing resilience and adapting to life's challenges with grace and determination. We offer insights into overcoming obstacles, managing setbacks, and maintaining a positive mindset even in the face of adversity.

By moving forward with confidence, individuals can embrace their newfound independence, discover their true potential, and create a life that aligns with their values and aspirations. This chapter serves as a guide to inspire and empower individuals as they embark on a journey of self-discovery, personal growth, and boundless possibilities.

Chapter 15: Embracing a Life of Resilience and Renewal

In the final chapter of Shattered Bonds, we explore the transformative journey of embracing a life of resilience and renewal after divorce. This chapter serves as a culmination of the lessons learned throughout the book, empowering individuals to rise above adversity and create a future filled with strength and renewal.

Within these pages, we delve into the importance of resilience as a powerful tool for navigating life's challenges. We provide insights into cultivating resilience through self-reflection, developing coping mechanisms, and embracing the lessons learned from the divorce experience.

This chapter addresses the significance of self-acceptance and letting go of regrets or lingering emotions from the past. We offer strategies for practicing forgiveness, both towards oneself and others, as a means of releasing emotional burdens and embracing a future free from resentment.

Additionally, we explore the potential for personal growth and self-discovery through embracing new opportunities and exploring uncharted paths. We discuss the importance of stepping outside of one's comfort zone, embracing change, and remaining open to the possibilities that life presents.

Furthermore, we discuss the importance of nurturing one's well-being holistically—mind, body, and soul. We provide guidance on self-care practices, healthy lifestyle choices, and cultivating a positive mindset that supports personal renewal and overall well-being.

In this chapter, we also address the significance of gratitude and finding joy in the present moment. We offer insights into cultivating a sense of appreciation for the blessings in life, practicing mindfulness, and savoring the simple pleasures that bring happiness and fulfillment.

By embracing a life of resilience and renewal, individuals can not only heal from the pain of divorce but also emerge stronger, wiser, and more resilient. This final chapter serves as a guide to inspire individuals to embrace their inner strength, embark on a path of personal renewal, and create a future that surpasses their wildest dreams.

Conclusion: Embracing a Journey of Healing and Growth

As we conclude our exploration of Shattered Bonds, we extend our heartfelt gratitude to you, the reader, for embarking on this transformative journey with us. We hope that the insights and guidance provided throughout this book have been a source of inspiration, comfort, and empowerment as you navigate the complexities of divorce and its aftermath.

Divorce is undoubtedly a challenging and emotional experience. However, we encourage you to remember that it is not the only option. We implore you to exhaust every possible avenue for reconciliation, seeking professional help, counseling, or mediation, before making the difficult decision to end a marriage.

Communication is the lifeblood of all relationships, and its significance cannot be overstated. It is through open and honest communication that misunderstandings can be resolved, conflicts can be addressed, and bonds can be strengthened. We urge you to prioritize communication in all your relationships, especially during times of hardship, as it lays the foundation for understanding, empathy, and growth.

Throughout the chapters of this book, we have explored the gamut of emotions that arise during divorce—grief, anger, sadness, and uncertainty. We have provided insights into healing emotional wounds, embracing change, and rediscovering oneself. We have offered guidance on co-

parenting, nurturing healthy relationships, and creating a vision
for the future.

Above all, we have emphasized the power of resilience, self-compassion, and personal growth. Divorce may mark the end of
a chapter, but it also presents an opportunity for new
beginnings and a chance to rewrite the narrative of your life.

We encourage you to approach this new chapter with courage,
grace, and a commitment to your own well-being. Embrace the
journey of healing and growth, knowing that you possess an
inner strength that can weather any storm. Seek support from
loved ones, professionals, and communities designed to uplift
and empower you.

Remember, you are not alone in this journey. Countless
individuals have navigated the path before you, and many more
will follow. Reach out, connect, and share your experiences. By
doing so, you contribute to a collective healing and inspire
others to find their own resilience.

Once again, we express our deepest gratitude for joining us on
this transformative exploration. May this book serve as a
beacon of hope, guidance, and encouragement as you embark
on a future filled with renewed strength, healing, and joy.

With warmest regards,

George Roberts

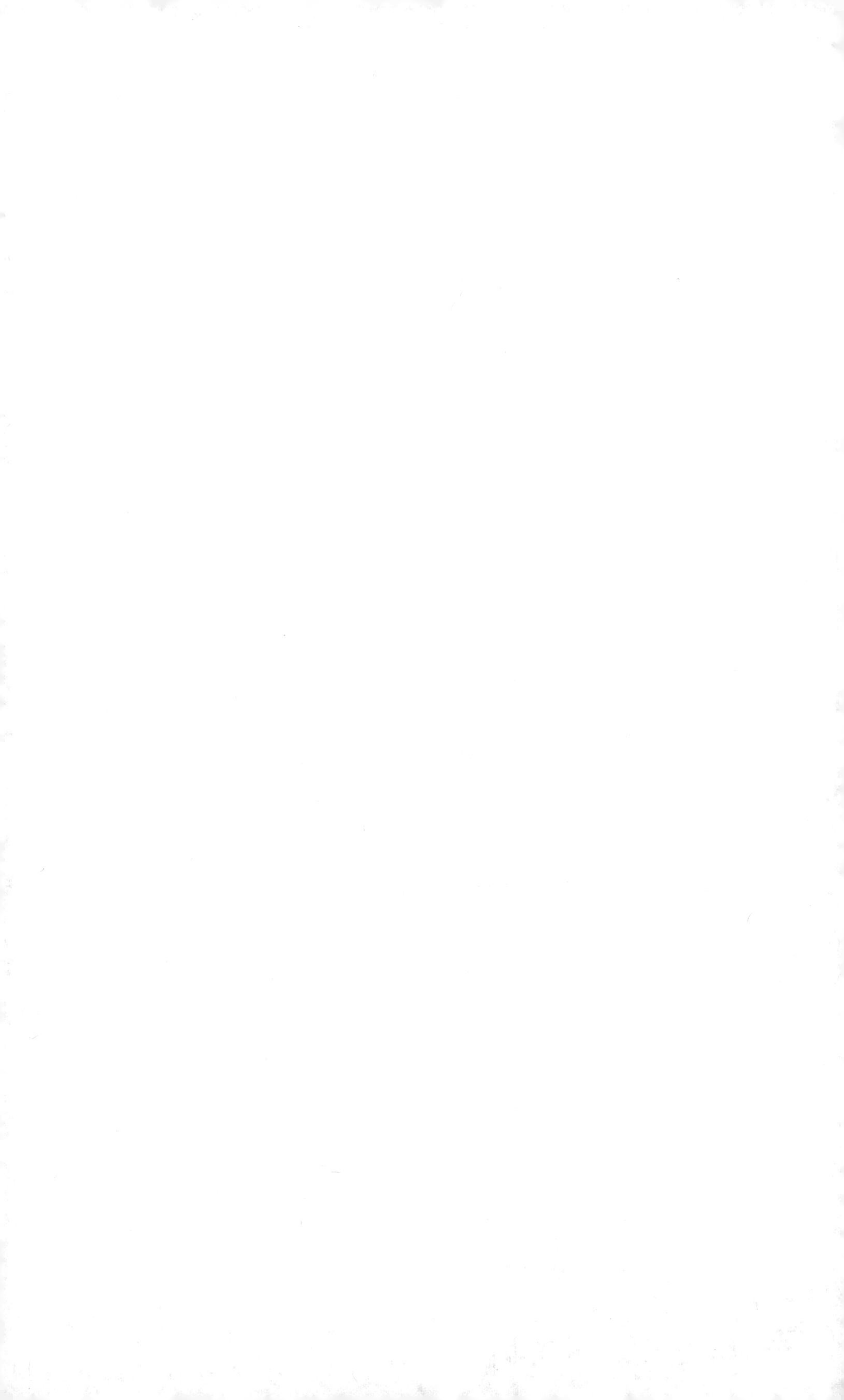